THE CANCER JOURNEY COMPANION

Book 1

Tips, Tools, and Strategies for Thriving Through Treatment

Evan K. Hayes

The information in this book is for educational purposes only. It is not intended to diagnose, treat, cure, or prevent any disease or medical condition. The author and publisher are not responsible for any adverse effects or consequences resulting from the use of the information contained in this book.

Table of Contents

INTRODUCTION

"Dave never expected to hear the word 'cancer' when he went in for a routine check-up. But as the doctor delivered the devastating news, Dave's world was turned upside down. Suddenly, he was faced with a daunting journey filled with chemotherapy, radiation, and surgeries. He didn't know where to turn or how to cope with the overwhelming physical and emotional challenges that lay ahead".

If you or a loved one have received a cancer diagnosis, it can be a scary and overwhelming time. You may feel unsure of where to turn or how to cope with the physical and emotional challenges of treatment. That's where The Cancer Journey Companion comes in.

This book, written by experts in cancer care, offers practical advice and strategies for managing the side effects of chemotherapy, communicating with healthcare providers, and finding support from loved ones. But it's not just about getting through treatment – it's about thriving. The book includes tips on how to maintain physical and emotional well-being, such as stress-reducing techniques, healthy eating habits, and exercise.

You don't have to face the cancer journey alone. The Cancer Journey Companion is a valuable resource that will be with you every step of the way, providing support and guidance as you navigate this difficult journey. Inside, you'll find valuable insights from experts and inspiring stories from cancer survivors. You'll learn how to manage your emotions, take care of yourself, and navigate the medical system.

The Cancer Journey Companion is more than just a book – it's a lifeline for anyone facing the challenges of cancer. If you or a loved one is going through a cancer diagnosis, don't hesitate to turn to this essential resource for the support and guidance you need to thrive.

CHAPTER ONE

Demystifying the Diagnosis: Understanding Your Cancer and Treatment Options

What is Cancer? Understanding the Basics

Cancer is a term used to describe a group of diseases that occur when cells in the body divide and grow in an uncontrolled way. Normally, our bodies can control the growth and division of cells through a process called cell cycle regulation. When this process goes awry, it can lead to the development of cancer.

There are many different types of cancer, each of which can develop in different parts of the body. Some common types of cancer include breast cancer, lung cancer, prostate cancer, and colon cancer. Cancer can also be classified by the type of cells it affects, such as carcinomas (cancers that affect the skin or the cells lining organs), sarcomas (cancers that affect connective tissue), or leukemias (cancers that affect the blood and bone marrow).

Cancer can be caused by a variety of factors, including genetic mutations, environmental exposures, and certain behaviors (such as tobacco use or excessive alcohol consumption). Some people may be at higher risk for developing cancer due to inherited genetic mutations or certain medical conditions, while others may be at higher risk due to their lifestyle or occupation.

There are many different ways to diagnose cancer, including physical exams, imaging tests (such as X-rays or CT scans), and biopsies. A biopsy is a procedure in which a small sample of tissue is taken from the affected area and examined under a microscope to determine if cancer cells are present.

Cancer is generally treated with a combination of surgery, chemotherapy, radiation therapy, or targeted therapies. The specific treatment approach will depend on the type and stage of cancer, as well as the individual's overall health and preferences.

It's important to note that cancer is a complex and often unpredictable disease, and every person's experience with cancer will be different. However, there are many resources available to help individuals and their families navigate the cancer journey, including support groups, patient advocacy organizations, and cancer centers. It's important to reach out for help and support whenever it is needed, as it can make a significant difference in managing the physical, emotional, and financial challenges that come with a cancer diagnosis.

The process of cancer development: Cancer begins when normal cells undergo a series of genetic mutations that allow them to grow and divide in an uncontrolled way. These abnormal cells can then form a mass, or tumor, which can grow and invade nearby tissues. In some cases, cancer cells can also spread, or metastasize, to other parts of the body through the bloodstream or lymphatic system. This process is known as metastasis.

Risk factors for cancer: Many factors can increase an individual's risk of developing cancer. Some of these include:

Age: The risk of developing cancer increases with age.

Genetics: Certain genetic mutations can increase the risk of developing cancer.

Lifestyle: Factors such as tobacco use, excessive alcohol consumption, unhealthy diet, and lack of exercise can increase the risk of cancer.

Environmental exposures: Exposure to certain chemicals or substances in the environment, such as radiation or certain types of infections, can increase the risk of cancer.

Medical conditions: Certain medical conditions, such as chronic inflammation or a weakened immune system, can increase the risk of cancer.

It's important to note that having one or more risk factors does not necessarily mean that an individual will develop cancer. Many people with several risk factors never develop the disease, while others with no known risk factors may be diagnosed with cancer.

Early detection and prevention: Early detection and prevention are key to improving outcomes for people with cancer. There are many screening tests available that can help detect cancer in its early stages when it is most treatable. Some common cancer screening tests include mammograms for breast cancer, colonoscopies for colon cancer, and prostate-specific antigen (PSA) tests for prostate cancer. In addition to screening tests, there are also many things that individuals can do to reduce their risk of developing cancer, such as quitting smoking, maintaining a healthy weight, and having a good and balanced diet amongst others.

Different types of cancer: Many different types of cancer can affect different parts of the body. Some of the most occurring types of cancer include:
Breast cancer: Breast cancer is the most occurring type of cancer in women. It occurs when cancer cells form in the tissue of the breast.

Lung cancer: Lung cancer is the leading cause of cancer-related deaths worldwide. It occurs when cancer cells form in the tissue of the lungs.

Prostate cancer: Prostate cancer is the most common type of cancer in men. It occurs when cancer cells form in the prostate, a gland in the male reproductive system.

Colon cancer: Colon cancer is cancer that affects the large intestine (colon) and rectum.

Leukemia: Leukemia is a cancer of the blood. It majorly affects the blood and bone marrow. It is characterized by the production of abnormal white blood cells.

Lymphoma: Lymphoma is a cancer that affects the immune system. It occurs when cancer cells form in the lymphatic system, a network of vessels and glands that help to fight infection.

Treatment options: There are many different treatment options available for cancer, including surgery, chemotherapy, radiation therapy, and targeted therapies. The specific treatment approach will depend on the type and stage of cancer, as well as the individual's overall health and preferences.

Surgery: Surgery is a common treatment option for cancer. It involves removing the cancerous tissue or organ to remove cancer from the body.

Chemotherapy: Chemotherapy is a treatment option that uses drugs to kill cancer cells. It can be administered orally or intravenously and may be used alone or in combination with other treatments.

Radiation therapy: Radiation therapy is a treatment option that uses high-energy beams of radiation to kill cancer cells. It can be administered externally (from a machine outside the body) or internally (using a device placed inside the body).

Targeted therapies: Targeted therapies are a type of treatment that focuses on specific genes or proteins that are involved in the development and growth of cancer cells.

These therapies can be used alone or in combination with other treatments.

Clinical trials: Clinical trials are research studies that test new treatments or approaches to cancer care. Participation in a clinical trial can provide access to cutting-edge treatments that are not yet widely available.

Your Diagnosis: What Does It Mean and What Comes Next?

Receiving a cancer diagnosis can be a frightening and overpowering experience. It's natural to have many questions and concerns about what the diagnosis means and what comes next. In this subchapter, we will explore some of the key issues that may arise after a cancer diagnosis.

Understanding your diagnosis: A cancer diagnosis generally includes information about the type and stage of cancer, as well as the available treatment options. It's important to understand this information to make informed decisions about your care.

Staging and grading: A cancer diagnosis often includes information about the stage and grade of cancer. The stage of cancer refers to the extent to which it has spread within the body. The higher the stage, the more advanced cancer. The grade of cancer refers to how abnormal the cancer cells look under a microscope and how quickly they are likely to grow and spread. Knowing the stage and grade of your cancer can help your healthcare team determine the most appropriate treatment approach.

Treatment goals: The goals of cancer treatment can vary depending on the type and stage of cancer, as well as the individual's overall health and preferences. Some common goals of cancer treatment include:

Cure: A cure is the complete removal of all cancer cells from the body. This is the goal of treatment for many types of cancer, especially when the cancer is caught in its early stages.

Control: In some cases, it may not be possible to completely cure cancer. In these situations, the goal of treatment may be to control cancer, either by slowing its growth or by keeping it in check.

Palliation: Palliation is the relief of symptoms caused by cancer. This may be the goal of treatment for people with advanced cancer or for those who are not candidates for curative treatment.

Side effects of treatment: Cancer treatment can cause a wide range of side effects, including fatigue, nausea, hair loss, and changes in appetite. It's important to discuss the potential side effects of treatment with your healthcare team and to work together to manage them. Many strategies can help reduce the impact of treatment side effects, including medications, lifestyle changes, and complementary therapies.

Follow-up care: Follow-up care is an important part of cancer treatment. It typically involves ongoing monitoring and management of cancer and any related health issues. Follow-up care may involve regular check-ups, imaging tests, and other procedures to ensure that the cancer is not returning and to identify any new health issues that may arise. It's important to follow the recommended follow-up care plan to ensure the best possible outcomes.

The importance of getting a second opinion: It's not uncommon for people to seek a second opinion after a cancer diagnosis. A second opinion can provide additional perspective and can be especially helpful if you're unsure about your treatment options or if you want to explore additional options. It's important to remember that it's okay to seek a second opinion, and in many cases, it can be a wise decision.

The role of a multidisciplinary team: Cancer treatment often involves a team of specialists who work together to provide comprehensive care. This team may include oncologists (doctors who specialize in cancer treatment), surgeons, radiation therapists, and other healthcare professionals. Working with a multidisciplinary team can help ensure that you receive the best possible care.

Treatment options: There are many different treatment options available for cancer, including surgery, chemotherapy, radiation therapy, and targeted therapies. The specific treatment approach will depend on the type and stage of cancer, as well as the individual's overall health and preferences. It's important to discuss all of your treatment options with your healthcare team and to consider factors such as the potential benefits and side effects of each option.

Clinical trials: Clinical trials are research studies that test new treatments or approaches to cancer care. Participation in a clinical trial can provide access to cutting-edge treatments that are not yet widely available. It's important to consider the potential benefits and risks of participating in a clinical trial and to discuss this option with your healthcare team.

Coping with a cancer diagnosis: A cancer diagnosis can be emotionally and physically challenging. It's important to take care of yourself and to seek support when you need it. This may involve seeking help from friends and family, participating in support groups, or working with a mental health professional.

Receiving a cancer diagnosis can be a difficult experience, but it's important to remember that you are not alone. There are many resources available to help you and your family navigate the cancer journey and to thrive through treatment.

Exploring Your Treatment Options: Pros and Cons

When it comes to cancer treatment, there are many options available. It's important to understand the pros and cons of each option to make an informed decision about your care. In this subchapter, we will explore some of the most common treatment options for cancer.

Surgery: Surgery is a common treatment option for cancer. It involves removing the cancerous tissue or organ to remove cancer from the body. Some of the pros of surgery include:

The ability to remove cancer: Surgery can be an effective treatment option for many types of cancer, especially when the cancer is caught in its early stages.

Relief of symptoms: In some cases, surgery can help relieve symptoms caused by cancer, such as pain or difficulty breathing.

Improved quality of life: Surgery can improve quality of life by restoring function or appearance.

Some of the cons of surgery include:

Risk of complications: Surgery carries a risk of complications, such as infection, bleeding, or scarring.

Recovery time: Surgery typically requires a period of recovery, which may involve pain and discomfort.

Potential for cosmetic changes: Depending on the type of surgery, there may be changes to appearance or function.

Chemotherapy: Chemotherapy is a treatment option that uses drugs to kill cancer cells. It can be administered orally or intravenously and may be used alone or in combination with other treatments. Some of the pros of chemotherapy include:
The ability to kill cancer cells: Chemotherapy can be an effective treatment option for many

types of cancer, especially when combined with other treatments.

Potential for improvement in symptoms: In some cases, chemotherapy can help improve symptoms caused by cancer, such as pain or shortness of breath.

Some of the cons of chemotherapy include:

Side effects: Chemotherapy can cause a wide range of side effects, including nausea, vomiting, hair loss, and fatigue.

Risk of infection: Chemotherapy can weaken the immune system, making it more difficult for the body to fight off infections.

Potential for long-term effects: Some chemotherapy drugs can have long-term effects on the body, including fertility issues and an increased risk of other health problems.

Radiation therapy: Radiation therapy is a treatment option that uses high-energy beams of radiation to kill cancer cells. It can be administered externally (from a machine outside the body) or internally (using a device placed inside the body). Some of the pros of radiation therapy include:

The ability to kill cancer cells: Radiation therapy can be an effective treatment option for many types of cancer, especially when combined with other treatments.

Relief of symptoms: In some cases, radiation therapy can help relieve symptoms caused by cancer, such as pain or difficulty swallowing.

Some of the cons of radiation therapy include:

Side effects: Radiation therapy can cause a wide range of side effects, including skin irritation, fatigue, and changes in appetite.

Risk of long-term effects: Some types of radiation therapy can have long-term effects on the body, including an increased risk of other health problems.

Limited to certain areas of the body: Radiation therapy is typically limited to certain areas of the body and may not be an option for cancers that have spread to multiple locations.

Targeted therapies: Targeted therapies are a type of treatment that focuses on specific genes or proteins that are involved in the development and growth of cancer cells. These therapies can be utilized on their own or in combination with other forms of treatment. Some of the pros of targeted therapies include:

Specificity: Targeted therapies are designed to specifically target cancer cells, which may help to minimize side effects.

Effectiveness: Some targeted therapies can be very effective at killing cancer cells, especially when used in combination with other treatments.

Some of the cons of targeted therapies include:

Limited effectiveness: While some targeted therapies can be very effective, others may be less so, depending on the specific cancer and the individual's unique situation.

Side effects: Targeted therapies can cause side effects, including skin rash, diarrhea, and changes in liver function.

Limited availability: Some targeted therapies are not yet widely available or may not be covered by insurance.

Clinical trials: Clinical trials are research studies that test new treatments or approaches to cancer care. Participation in a clinical trial can provide access to cutting-edge treatments that are not yet widely available. Some of the pros of participating in a clinical trial include:

Access to innovative treatments: Clinical trials provide an opportunity to try treatments that are not yet widely available.

Contribution to scientific knowledge: Participation in a clinical trial can contribute to the advancement of cancer research and may lead to new and better treatments in the future.

Close monitoring: Clinical trials often involve close monitoring by a team of healthcare professionals, which can provide additional support and care.

Some of the cons of participating in a clinical trial include:

Risk of unknown side effects: Clinical trials involve testing new treatments, which means that the potential side effects may not be fully known.

Limited availability: Clinical trials may not be available in all areas or may have strict eligibility criteria.

Time and logistical considerations: Participation in a clinical trial may require additional time and logistical considerations, such as traveling to appointments or taking additional medications.

It's important to carefully consider the pros and cons of each treatment option and to discuss your options with your healthcare team. Ultimately, the decision about which treatment approach is best will depend on your circumstances, including the type and stage of cancer, your overall health, and your preference

CHAPTER TWO

Building a Support Team: How to Find and Lean on Loved Ones During Treatment

Identifying your support needs: A self-assessment guide

As a cancer patient, it is important to identify your support needs and build a team of loved ones who can help you during treatment. This process can be overwhelming, especially if you are a first-time patient, but it is essential to take the time to carefully consider your needs and how they may change throughout your treatment.

One way to begin this process is to complete a self-assessment of your support needs. This can help you to identify the areas where you may need the most help and will allow you to communicate your needs more effectively to your loved ones. Here are some questions to consider as you complete your self-assessment:

What tasks do you need help with? This could include things like transportation to and from appointments, grocery shopping, and household chores.

Who do you feel most comfortable talking to about your feelings and experiences? This could be a family member, a close friend, or a mental health professional.

What type of emotional support do you need? This could include things like listening, reassurance, or simply being present.

What is your preferred method of communication with loved ones? Some people prefer phone calls, text messages, or in-person visits, while others may prefer written communication or online chat.

As you complete your self-assessment, be sure, to be honest with yourself about your needs. It is important to remember that it is okay to ask for help and that you do not have to go through this journey alone. Your loved ones are there to support you, and it is important to be open and honest with them about what you need.

Once you have completed your self-assessment, you can begin to identify the people in your life who can best meet your needs. This may include family members, friends, and professionals, such as doctors, nurses, and therapists. It is important to choose people who are reliable, understanding, and willing to be there for you during this challenging time.

Remember, your support team does not have to be limited to just a few people. You may find that you need different types of support from different people at different times. It is okay to seek support from multiple sources and to ask for help when you need it.

Overall, the key to building a strong support team is to be open and honest about your needs and to choose people who are reliable and willing to be there for you. With the right team in place, you will be better equipped to navigate the challenges of cancer treatment and thrive during this difficult time.

Assembling your dream team: How to choose the right people for your support network

As you begin to build your support team, it is important to choose people who are reliable, understanding, and able to meet your needs. Here are some tips to help you choose the right people for your support network:

Consider your needs: As you identified in your self-assessment, think about the specific tasks and emotional support that you need. Look for people who can provide the specific support that you need.

Be honest and open: Be upfront about your needs and expectations with the people you are considering for your support team. This will help to ensure that everyone is on the same page and that you are getting the support you need.

Don't be afraid to ask for help: It can be difficult to ask for help, but it is important to remember that your loved ones are there to support you. Don't be afraid to ask for the help you need, whether it is for practical tasks or emotional support.

Be selective: It is okay to be selective about who you include on your support team. You don't have to include everyone who offers to help. Choose the people who you feel most comfortable with and who can meet your needs.

Once you have identified the people you want to include on your support team, it is important to communicate your needs and expectations. Let your loved ones know how they can best support you and what you need from them. This may include things like making sure you have transportation to appointments, helping with household chores, or simply being available to listen and provide emotional support.

Remember, your support team does not have to be limited to just a few people. You may find that you need different types of support from different people at different times. It is okay to seek support from multiple sources and to ask for help when you need it.

It is also important to keep in mind that your support needs may change throughout your treatment. You may find that you need more support at certain times than others, or that your needs change as your treatment progresses. Be sure to communicate any changes in your needs to your support team so that they can continue to meet your needs effectively.

In addition to friends and family, there are also many professional resources available to help you during your cancer journey. These may include doctors, nurses, therapists, and social workers. These professionals can provide medical care, emotional support, and practical assistance to help you navigate the challenges of cancer treatment.

If you are having difficulty finding the support you need, there are also many cancer support groups and organizations that can provide additional resources and support. These groups can be a great source of information and can help connect you with others who are going through similar experiences.

Overall, building a strong support team is essential for thriving during cancer treatment. By carefully choosing the right people and being open and honest about your needs, you can create a team that will be there for you every step of the way. Don't be afraid to seek out additional resources and support if you need it, and remember that it is okay to ask for help when you need it. With the right support in place, you can feel more confident and capable of facing the challenges of cancer treatment.

Maximizing support from friends and family: Practical tips for communicating your needs and setting boundaries

Once you have assembled your support team, it is important to effectively communicate your needs and set boundaries to ensure that you are getting the support you need. Here are some practical tips for maximizing support from your loved ones:

Communicate clearly: Be specific about what you need and how your loved ones can help. Don't be afraid to ask for specific tasks or types of support.

Set boundaries: It is important to set boundaries to protect your time, energy, and well-being. This may include setting limits on how much time you are willing to spend on the phone or in person with loved ones, or asking for privacy when you need it.

Be open and honest: Don't be afraid to share your feelings and experiences with your loved ones. This can help to strengthen your relationships and provide you with the emotional support you need.

Seek support from multiple sources: Don't rely on just one or two people for all of your support. It is okay to seek support from multiple sources, including friends, family, professionals, and support groups.

It is also important to remember that your loved ones may need support as well. Being a caregiver can be emotionally and physically demanding, and it is important to ensure that your loved ones are taking care of themselves as well. Encourage your loved ones to seek their support and to set their boundaries as needed.

It is also helpful to be flexible and open to trying new forms of support. Your loved ones may have different ideas about how to best support you, and it is important to be open to trying new things. For example, your loved ones may suggest using technology to stay in touch, such as video calls or online chat. These forms of communication can be a convenient and effective way to stay connected, especially if you are unable to meet in person due to treatment or other commitments.

It is also important to remember that your support needs may change over time. As your treatment progresses, your needs may shift, and it is important to communicate these changes to your loved ones so that they can continue to support you effectively.

Finally, don't be afraid to seek professional support if you need it. Mental health professionals, such as therapists and social workers, can provide additional support and can help you to manage the emotional challenges of cancer treatment. These professionals can also help you to communicate your needs effectively to your loved ones and to set boundaries as needed.

Overall, maximizing support from friends and family is essential for thriving during cancer treatment. By being open and honest about your needs, setting boundaries, and seeking professional support as needed, you can ensure that you have the support you need to navigate the challenges of cancer treatment and thrive during this difficult time.

CHAPTER THREE

Coping with the Emotional Rollercoaster: Strategies for Managing Your Mood and Mindset

Navigating the ups and downs: Tips for managing the emotional highs and lows of cancer treatment

As a cancer patient, it's common to experience a wide range of emotions during treatment. These emotions can be intense and may come and go quickly, leading to what can feel like an emotional rollercoaster. It's important to remember that it's normal to feel this way and that there are strategies you can use to help manage your emotions during this time.

One tip for managing the emotional ups and downs of cancer treatment is to allow yourself to feel your emotions. It's important to acknowledge and validate your feelings, rather than trying to push them away or ignore them. This can help you better understand and cope with what you're going through.

It's also helpful to find healthy ways to express your emotions. This might include talking with a loved one, writing in a journal, or finding a creative outlet like art or music.

It can also be helpful to set aside time to practice self-care. This might include activities like exercise, meditation, or getting enough sleep. Taking care of your physical and emotional well-being can help you feel more grounded and better equipped to handle the challenges of cancer treatment.

Another strategy for managing the emotional ups and downs of cancer treatment is to seek support from loved ones and professional resources. This might include talking with a therapist, joining a support group, or connecting with other cancer survivors. Having a strong support system can provide a sense of comfort and help you feel less alone during this difficult time.

It's also important to remember that it's acceptable to request assistance. Don't be afraid to lean on loved ones for emotional support, or to seek out professional resources if you need additional support.

Overall, managing the emotional ups and downs of cancer treatment can be challenging, but there are strategies you can use to help cope with these emotions. By allowing yourself to feel your emotions, finding healthy ways to express them, practicing self-care, and seeking support, you can better navigate the emotional rollercoaster of cancer treatment.

Finding support: How to connect with loved ones and professional resources during treatment

Cancer treatment can be an emotionally and physically draining experience. It's natural to feel overwhelmed, anxious, and isolated during this time. Having a strong support system can make a significant difference in your ability to cope with the challenges of treatment. Here, we will explore ways to connect with loved ones and professional resources to help you build a supportive network.

Connecting with Loved Ones

Reaching out to loved ones is an important aspect of finding support during cancer treatment. It can be difficult to ask for help, especially if you're feeling vulnerable or unsure of how to do so. However, it's important to remember that your loved ones want to be there for you and are likely willing to do whatever they can to support you. Consider having a conversation with your family and close friends to let them know how they can help. This can include offering practical support, such as helping with household chores or transportation to appointments, or simply being a listening ear when you need to talk.

Connecting with Professional Resources

In addition to reaching out to loved ones, it can also be helpful to connect with professional resources. This can include seeking out a cancer support group or joining an online community of people who are also going through cancer treatment. These types of resources can provide a sense of community and can be a helpful way to connect with others who are experiencing similar emotions and challenges.

Another option is to talk to a mental health professional, such as a therapist or counselor. These professionals can provide a safe and confidential space for you to process your emotions and learn coping strategies to manage the challenges of cancer treatment. They can also help you identify and address any underlying mental health issues that may be exacerbating your stress and anxiety.

It's important to remember that finding support is a personal journey and what works for one person may not work for another. It may take some trial and error to figure out what works best for you, but don't be afraid to reach out and ask for help. Building a supportive network can make a huge difference in your ability to thrive during treatment.

Creating a positive mindset: Strategies for maintaining a hopeful and resilient attitude during treatment

Maintaining a positive mindset can be a powerful tool for coping with the challenges of cancer treatment. Research has shown that people who approach their treatment with a hopeful and resilient attitude are more likely to experience better physical and emotional outcomes. In this sub-chapter, we will explore strategies for creating and maintaining a positive mindset during treatment.

One of the key strategies for maintaining a positive mindset is to focus on the things you can control. Cancer treatment can be unpredictable and it's natural to feel a sense of loss of control. However, focusing on the things you can control, such as your diet, exercise routine, and stress management techniques, can help you feel more in control of your situation. It can also be helpful to set small, achievable goals for yourself to help you feel a sense of progress and accomplishment.

Another important strategy is to cultivate a sense of gratitude. This can involve taking the time to appreciate the good things in your life, no matter how small they may seem. This could be something as simple as enjoying a cup of coffee or spending time with loved ones. Focusing on the positive can help you stay hopeful and resilient, even when things feel difficult.

It's also important to find healthy ways to manage stress and emotions. This could include activities like exercise, mindfulness practices, or talking to a mental health professional. Taking care of your emotional well-being can help you maintain a positive mindset and better cope with the challenges of treatment.

Finally, it's important to remember that it's okay to have moments of negativity and sadness. It's a normal part of the cancer journey and it's important to give yourself permission to feel and express your emotions. However, by focusing on strategies like those mentioned above, you can cultivate a more hopeful and resilient attitude that will help you thrive during treatment.

CHAPTER FOUR

Navigating the Medical Maze: Tips for Communicating with Your Healthcare Team and Getting the Care You Need

The cancer journey can be overwhelming and it can be difficult to navigate the complex world of healthcare. In Chapter Four of THE CANCER JOURNEY COMPANION, we will explore tips for communicating with your healthcare team and getting the care you need. Effective communication with your healthcare team is crucial for ensuring that your needs and concerns are heard and addressed. We will also delve into strategies for managing insurance and financial considerations, including understanding your insurance coverage, exploring financial assistance options, and negotiating costs. By following these tips and strategies, you can take an active role in your care and feel more in control of your cancer journey.

Building a strong healthcare team: How to find and choose the right doctors and specialists for your treatment journey

Building a strong healthcare team is an important aspect of your cancer journey. The right team can provide you with the support and care you need to navigate your treatment and manage any side effects or other challenges that may arise. Here are some tips for finding and choosing the right doctors and specialists for your treatment journey:

Start with your primary care physician: Your primary care physician is your first point of contact for your healthcare needs and can help coordinate your care with specialists. If you don't have a primary care physician, or if your current one is not familiar with cancer treatment, consider finding one who is.

Seek out specialists: Depending on the type and stage of your cancer, you may need to see a variety of specialists, such as a medical oncologist, radiation oncologist, and/or surgical oncologist. Ask your primary care physician for recommendations, or consider getting a second opinion from another specialist.

Consider the team's experience: Look for doctors and specialists who have experience treating your specific type of cancer. Ask about their success rates and treatment approaches.

Check their credentials: Make sure the doctors and specialists you are considering are licensed and board-certified in their respective fields. You can check their credentials by looking up their names on the American Medical Association's website or by asking the hospital or clinic where they work.

Consider the location: You may need to see your healthcare team frequently during your treatment, so it's important to choose doctors and specialists who are conveniently located. Consider factors like distance from your home or work, and whether the location has good public transportation options.

Think about communication style: It's important that you feel comfortable communicating with your healthcare team. Consider whether you prefer doctors who are more directive or those who are more collaborative. You should also consider whether the team communicates well with each other and whether they are willing to listen to your concerns and answer your questions.

Take your time: Don't feel rushed to decide on your healthcare team. Take the time to research your options and talk to multiple doctors and specialists before making a decision. You may also want to consult with friends, family, or support groups to get additional perspectives.

By following these tips, you can build a strong healthcare team that will provide you with the support and cares you need to thrive during your cancer journey.

Effective communication with your healthcare team: Tips for expressing your needs and concerns

Effective communication with your healthcare team is crucial for ensuring that you receive the best possible care during your cancer journey. It can be intimidating to speak up and advocate for yourself, especially when you are dealing with a serious illness. However, it is important to remember that your healthcare team is there to support you and help you through this difficult time. By learning how to effectively communicate with your healthcare team, you can ensure that your needs and concerns are heard and addressed.

Here are some tips for expressing your needs and concerns to your healthcare team:

Be clear and concise: It can be overwhelming to try to convey all of your thoughts and feelings at once. Instead, focus on expressing one main concern or question at a time. This will help your healthcare team better understand your needs and provide more targeted support.

Don't be afraid to ask questions: It is completely normal to have questions and concerns about your treatment and care. Your healthcare team is there to help you, so don't be afraid to ask questions. If you don't understand something, ask for clarification. It is better to ask and receive a clear explanation than to be left in the dark.

Use "I" statements: When expressing your needs and concerns, try to use "I" statements rather than "you" statements. For example, instead of saying "you're not listening to me," try saying "I feel like my concerns are not being heard." This approach is more respectful and less confrontational, and it can help facilitate better communication with your healthcare team.

Bring a support person: It can be helpful to bring a family member or friend to your appointments to provide emotional support and to help you communicate your needs and concerns. This person can also help you remember important information and ask questions that you may not have thought of.

Write things down: It can be helpful to bring a notebook or a list of questions and concerns to your appointments. This can help you stay organized and ensure that you don't forget anything important. It can also be helpful to bring copies of your medical records and any test results to your appointments so that your healthcare team has all of the information they need to make informed decisions about your care.

Effective communication with your healthcare team is an important part of your cancer journey. By expressing your needs and concerns, you can ensure that you receive the best possible care and support during this difficult time.

Navigating insurance and financial considerations: Strategies for getting the care you need while managing costs

Managing insurance and financial considerations can be a daunting task during your cancer journey. It is important to remember that your healthcare team is there to support you and help you navigate these challenges. Here are some strategies for getting the care you need while managing costs:

Understand your insurance coverage: It is important to understand your insurance coverage and what is covered under your plan. This includes things like doctor visits, tests, and treatments. Be sure to read your insurance policy and ask your healthcare team or insurance provider any questions you may have.

Look into financial assistance programs: Many hospitals and cancer centers offer financial assistance programs to help patients with the cost of treatment. These programs can assist with things like copays, deductibles, and other out-of-pocket expenses. Be sure to ask your healthcare team about financial assistance options.

Explore other payment options: If you are struggling to afford your treatment, you may be able to negotiate a payment plan with your healthcare provider. This can allow you to pay for your treatment over time rather than upfront. You may also be able to use a credit card or take out a loan to cover the cost of your treatment.

Consider clinical trials: Clinical trials are research studies that test new treatments for a variety of medical conditions. Some clinical trials offer free treatment to participants, and they can be a good option for patients who are struggling to afford their care. However, it is important to carefully consider the potential risks and benefits of participating in a clinical trial before making a decision.

Don't be afraid to ask for help: Managing the financial aspects of your cancer journey can be overwhelming. Don't be afraid to ask for help from your healthcare team, social worker, or financial counselor. They can provide you with resources and support to help you navigate these challenges.

In addition to the strategies mentioned above, here are a few more tips for managing insurance and financial considerations during your cancer journey:

Keep track of your expenses: It can be helpful to keep track of your medical expenses, including things like copays, deductibles, and any out-of-pocket expenses. This can help you stay organized and understand your financial situation.

Review your bills carefully: Make sure to review your medical bills carefully, as mistakes and errors can sometimes occur. If you notice any discrepancies, be sure to contact your healthcare provider or insurance company to resolve them.

Check for billing errors: It is not uncommon for medical billing errors to occur, so it is important to carefully review your bills for any mistakes. If you notice any errors, be sure to report them to your healthcare provider or insurance company as soon as possible.

Negotiate your costs: If you are struggling to afford your treatment, you may be able to negotiate the cost with your healthcare provider. This can include things like lower copays or deductibles, or a reduced price for medications or treatments. Don't be afraid to ask your healthcare team or insurance company if there are any options for lowering your costs.

Consider crowdfunding: Crowdfunding is a way to raise money for a specific cause or project through small donations from a large number of people. If you are struggling to afford your treatment, you may be able to use crowdfunding to cover your medical expenses. Several online platforms allow you to create a campaign and share your story with potential donors.

Managing insurance and financial considerations is a critical part of your cancer journey. By understanding your insurance coverage, exploring financial assistance options, and seeking help when needed, you can ensure that you receive the care you need while managing costs.

CHAPTER FIVE

Eating for Healing: The Importance of Nutrition During Cancer Treatment

As you embark on your cancer journey, one important aspect of your care will be your nutrition. While it may not be the first thing on your mind during treatment, the food you eat can have a significant impact on your overall health and well-being. In this chapter, we will explore the importance of nutrition during cancer treatment, and provide tips, tools, and strategies for thriving through treatment by eating for healing. Whether you are dealing with appetite changes, dietary restrictions, or treatment-related side effects, we will provide practical guidance on how to nourish your body and support your healing process. By making mindful and nourishing choices, you can take an active role in your recovery and feel your best during this challenging time.

The role of nutrition in cancer treatment

Nutrition plays a crucial role in cancer treatment, as it can affect both the effectiveness of treatment and a person's overall quality of life. Good nutrition can help the body to recover from treatment, maintain strength and energy, and prevent infection and other complications. Poor nutrition, on the other hand, can weaken the body, making it more vulnerable to infection and other problems.

There is evidence to suggest that proper nutrition can also improve treatment outcomes. For example, research has shown that people with cancer who maintain a healthy weight and consume a balanced diet may be more likely to respond well to treatment and have a better prognosis. Similarly, people who are undernourished or have poor nutritional status may be at higher risk for treatment-related side effects and complications.

Given the importance of nutrition in cancer treatment, it is essential for people with cancer to pay close attention to their diet and make sure they are getting all the nutrients they need. This may involve working with a nutritionist or dietitian to develop a customized meal plan, as well as seeking support from friends and family to ensure that nutritional needs are met.

Here are some key considerations for maintaining good nutrition during cancer treatment:

Maintaining a healthy weight: Cancer treatment can cause changes in appetite and metabolism that may affect weight. Some people may lose weight due to treatment-related side effects such as nausea, vomiting, or decreased appetite. Others may gain weight due to treatment-related changes in metabolism or due to an increase in appetite. It is important to aim for a healthy weight and to work with a healthcare team to manage any changes in weight during treatment.

Consuming a balanced diet: A balanced diet is essential for maintaining good nutrition during cancer treatment. This means eating a variety of foods from all food groups, including proteins, carbohydrates, fats, fruits, vegetables, and fluids. It is important to choose nutrient-rich foods that provide the energy and nutrients the body needs to heal and recover.

Managing treatment-related side effects: Treatment-related side effects, such as nausea, vomiting, mouth sores, and taste changes, can make it difficult to eat and drink enough to meet nutritional needs. It is important to work with a healthcare team to manage these side effects and to seek support from a nutritionist or dietitian to develop strategies for maintaining good nutrition.

Seeking support: Cancer treatment can be overwhelming, and it is natural to feel anxious or depressed at times. It is important to seek support from friends, family, and healthcare professionals to help manage the emotional and physical challenges of treatment. This may include seeking support from a nutritionist or dietitian to develop a meal plan that meets nutritional needs and addresses any challenges with eating and drinking.

By paying attention to nutrition during cancer treatment, you can support your body's healing process and improve your quality of life.

The importance of a balanced diet during treatment

A balanced diet is essential for maintaining good nutrition during cancer treatment. This means eating a variety of foods from all food groups, including proteins, carbohydrates, fats, fruits, vegetables, and fluids. Each food group provides different nutrients that are important for good health, and it is important to consume a mix of these nutrients to support the body's healing process.

Proteins are an important nutrient for people with cancer, as they help to repair and rebuild tissues, maintain muscle mass, and boost the immune system. Good sources of protein include meat, poultry, fish, beans, nuts, and dairy products. It is important to choose high-quality proteins that are rich in essential amino acids, as these are the building blocks of protein that the body needs to function properly.

Carbohydrates are another essential nutrient that provides the body with energy. They are found in a variety of foods, including grains, fruits, vegetables, and dairy products. It is important to choose complex carbohydrates, such as whole grains, beans, and vegetables, as these provide the body with sustained energy and are rich in fiber, vitamins, and minerals. Simple carbohydrates, such as sugar, should be consumed in moderation, as they can provide a quick burst of energy but may cause blood sugar levels to fluctuate.

Fats are an important source of energy and are essential for maintaining healthy skin, hair, and nails. They also help to absorb fat-soluble vitamins and minerals, such as vitamins A, D, E, and K. There are different types of fats, including saturated, monounsaturated, and polyunsaturated fats. It is important to choose healthy fats, such as olive oil, avocado, and nuts, and to limit your intake of unhealthy fats, such as trans fats and saturated fats.

Fruits and vegetables are important sources of vitamins, minerals, and antioxidants, which help to support the immune system and protect against disease. It is important to consume a variety of fruits and vegetables, as each one provides a unique mix of nutrients. It is also important to choose fresh, whole foods rather than processed or packaged foods, as these tend to be lower in nutrients and higher in additives and preservatives.

Fluids are essential for maintaining hydration and are important for maintaining good health during cancer treatment. It is important to consume adequate fluids, especially during treatment, as chemotherapy and other treatments can cause dehydration. Water is the best source of hydration, but other fluids, such as juices, soups, and smoothies, can also contribute to fluid intake. It is important to avoid sugary drinks, as these can contribute to weight gain and other health problems.

By consuming a balanced diet during cancer treatment, you can support your body's healing process and maintain good health. It is important to work with a healthcare team, including a nutritionist or dietitian, to develop a meal plan that meets your nutritional needs and addresses any challenges with eating and drinking. With careful planning and support, you can nourish your body and support your healing journey.

Managing chemotherapy-induced nausea and vomiting through diet

Chemotherapy-induced nausea and vomiting (CINV) is a common side effect of chemotherapy that can affect a person's appetite, nutrition, and overall quality of life. CINV occurs when chemotherapy drugs irritate the lining of the stomach and intestines, causing nausea and vomiting. It can also be caused by the brain's reaction to chemotherapy, which can cause the body to produce excess stomach acid or cause the muscles in the intestines to contract excessively.

CINV can be managed through a combination of medications and dietary strategies. It is important to work with a healthcare team to develop a plan to manage CINV, as each person's experience with CINV is unique.

Here are some dietary strategies that may help to manage CINV during chemotherapy:

Eat small, frequent meals: Eating smaller, more frequent meals may be easier on the stomach and help to prevent nausea. It is also important to choose foods that are easy to digest, such as broth-based soups, cooked vegetables, and cooked grains.

Avoid strong smells: Strong smells can trigger nausea and vomiting, so it may be helpful to avoid foods with strong odors, such as spicy foods, onions, and garlic.

Eat cold or room temperature foods: Hot foods may be more likely to trigger nausea and vomiting, so it may be helpful to eat cold or room temperature foods, such as cold sandwiches or smoothies.

Sip fluids slowly: Sipping fluids slowly may help to prevent dehydration and may also help to ease nausea. It is important to drink fluids that are clear or pale yellow, such as water, broth, and sports drinks, as these are easier on the stomach.

Avoid foods that are high in fat: High-fat foods can be more difficult to digest and may trigger nausea and vomiting. It is important to choose low-fat foods, such as lean proteins, cooked vegetables, and whole grains.

Eat foods that are high in protein: Protein is an important nutrient for maintaining muscle mass and supporting the immune system, and it may also help to manage CINV. Good sources of protein include meat, poultry, fish, beans, nuts, and dairy products.

It is important to work with a healthcare team to manage CINV during chemotherapy, as each person's experience with CINV is unique. In addition to dietary strategies, medications may also be used to manage CINV. These may include anti-nausea medications, which can help to prevent nausea and vomiting, and anti-emetic medications, which can help to control nausea and vomiting once it has started.

By following a healthy diet and seeking support from a healthcare team, it is possible to manage CINV and maintain good nutrition during chemotherapy.

CHAPTER SIX

Staying Active and Engaged: The Role of Exercise and Hobbies in Your Recovery

Welcome to Chapter Six of The Cancer Journey Companion: Staying Active and Engaged. In this chapter, we will explore the role of exercise and hobbies in your recovery from cancer. Exercise and hobbies can be powerful tools in helping you maintain physical and mental well-being during treatment and beyond. They can also provide a sense of purpose and a way to engage with the world around you. In this chapter, we will discuss the benefits of exercise and hobbies for cancer survivors, offer tips for finding and maintaining an active and engaged lifestyle, and provide resources for further support. Whether you are just beginning your cancer journey or are well into your recovery, we hope this chapter will provide you with the information and inspiration you need to stay active and engaged.

The Benefits of Exercise During Cancer Treatment: How physical activity can help manage treatment side effects, boost energy levels, and improve overall health and well-being.

Exercise and physical activity can be an important part of cancer treatment and recovery. While it may not be the first thing that comes to mind when faced with a cancer diagnosis, staying active and engaged through exercise and hobbies can provide a range of physical and mental health benefits.

One of the main benefits of exercise during cancer treatment is that it can help manage side effects and improve overall health and well-being. Cancer treatment can take a toll on the body, causing fatigue, weight gain, muscle loss, and other side effects. Exercise can help counteract these effects by boosting energy levels, improving muscle strength and endurance, and helping with weight management.

Exercise can also help reduce the risk of developing other health conditions, such as heart disease, diabetes, and osteoporosis, which may be more common in cancer survivors. In addition, research has shown that regular physical activity can improve mood, reduce stress and anxiety, and improve sleep quality, which can be especially important during cancer treatment.

It's important to keep in mind that the type and intensity of exercise should be tailored to your individual needs and abilities. It's always a good idea to consult with your healthcare team before starting an exercise program, especially if you have any underlying medical conditions or are currently undergoing treatment.

During cancer treatment, it's important to choose activities that are safe and enjoyable. This may include low-impact activities such as walking, swimming, or yoga, or more strenuous activities such as weight lifting or cycling, depending on your fitness level and goals. It's also important to listen to your body and not push yourself too hard. It's okay to take breaks and rest when needed.

In addition to exercise, hobbies can also play a role in helping you stay active and engaged during cancer treatment. Engaging in activities that bring you joy and a sense of accomplishment can help boost your mood and provide a sense of purpose. This might include hobbies such as painting, gardening, cooking, or playing a musical instrument.

Overall, the benefits of exercise and hobbies during cancer treatment are numerous. Staying active and engaged can help manage treatment side effects, boost energy levels, and improve overall health and well-being. It's important to consult with your healthcare team before starting an exercise program and choose activities that are safe and enjoyable. So, it is always better to stay active and engaged to maintain a healthy lifestyle.

Finding the Right Exercise for You: Tips for selecting activities that are safe and enjoyable, such as walking, swimming, or cycling.

Finding the right exercise for you during cancer treatment is important for managing side effects and improving overall health and well-being. Here are some tips for selecting activities that are safe and enjoyable:

Consult with your healthcare team: Before starting any exercise program, it's important to consult with your healthcare team to ensure that it is safe for you. Your healthcare team can guide the types and intensity of exercise that are appropriate for you based on your individual needs and abilities.

Choose activities that you enjoy: It's important to choose activities that you find enjoyable, as this will make it more likely that you will stick with them. This might include low-impact activities such as walking, swimming, or yoga, or more strenuous activities such as weight lifting or cycling.

Start slowly and gradually increase intensity: If you are new to exercise or have not been active for a while, it's important to start slowly and gradually increase the intensity of your workouts. This will allow your body to adapt and reduce the risk of injury.

Pay attention to your body and be mindful of not overexerting yourself. It's okay to take breaks and rest when needed. If you are experiencing any discomfort or pain, it's important to stop and consult with your healthcare team.

Consider working with a personal trainer or exercise coach: If you are unsure about how to get started with exercise or have any specific goals, consider working with a personal trainer or exercise coach. They can offer guidance and support to assist you in achieving your goals safely and effectively.

Overall, it's important to find an exercise program that is safe and enjoyable for you. By following these tips and consulting with your healthcare team, you can find the right exercise program to help you thrive during cancer treatment.

Overcoming Exercise Barriers: Strategies for overcoming common obstacles to physical activity, such as fatigue, pain, or lack of motivation.

It can be challenging to stay active and engaged during cancer treatment, and there may be several obstacles that can stand in the way of getting regular exercise. Here are some strategies for overcoming common barriers to physical activity:

Plan: To help overcome fatigue and lack of motivation, try to plan your workouts and schedule them into your day. This can help you stay on track and make it more likely that you will follow through with your exercise routine.

Make it convenient: Choose activities that are convenient and easy to fit into your daily routine. For example, if you have limited energy or mobility, consider activities that can be done at home or in your local community.

Find a workout buddy: Having a workout buddy can provide motivation and accountability, and make exercise more enjoyable. You could ask a friend or family member to join you, or consider joining a group exercise class or online workout group.

Focus on the benefits: It can be helpful to remind yourself of the benefits of exercise, such as improved energy levels, mood, and overall health and well-being. This can help motivate you to get moving, even on days when you don't feel like it.

Modify your workouts: If you are experiencing pain or discomfort, try modifying your workouts or choosing low-impact activities that are easier on your body. You could also consider working with a physical therapist or exercise coach to help you find safe and effective ways to stay active.

Overall, it's important to find strategies that work for you to overcome common barriers to physical activity during cancer treatment. By planning, making exercise convenient, finding a workout buddy, focusing on the benefits, and modifying your workouts as needed, you can stay active and engaged despite the challenges.

Engaging in Hobbies and Leisure Activities: Ideas for finding joy and purpose through hobbies and leisure activities, such as gardening, painting, or reading.

Hobbies and leisure activities can be an important part of cancer treatment and recovery, providing a sense of joy and purpose and helping to boost mood and well-being. Here are some ideas for finding hobbies and leisure activities that bring you enjoyment and a sense of accomplishment:

Reflect on your interests and passions: Take some time to think about what you enjoy doing in your free time. This could include activities such as gardening, painting, cooking, reading, or playing a musical instrument.

Experiment with different activities: Don't be afraid to try new things and see what works for you. You may discover a new hobby or activity that brings you joy and a sense of accomplishment.

Find ways to engage in your hobbies and leisure activities safely: During cancer treatment, it's important to choose activities that are safe and enjoyable. This might mean finding ways to modify your hobbies or leisure activities to make them easier on your body. For example, if you enjoy gardening but have limited mobility, you could consider container gardening or working in raised beds.

Seek out supportive resources and communities: There are many resources and communities available to support people with cancer in finding and engaging in hobbies and leisure activities. These might include cancer support groups, online communities, or local organizations that offer classes or workshops.

Overall, hobbies and leisure activities can be an important part of cancer treatment and recovery, providing a sense of joy and purpose and helping to boost mood and well-being. By reflecting on your interests and passions, experimenting with different activities, finding ways to engage in your hobbies safely, and seeking out supportive resources and communities, you can find ways to stay active and engaged through hobbies and leisure activities during cancer treatment.

Staying Active and Engaged After Treatment: Strategies for maintaining an active lifestyle

and continuing to engage in hobbies and leisure activities after treatment is completed.

Maintaining an active lifestyle and continuing to engage in hobbies and leisure activities after cancer treatment is an important aspect of cancer recovery and overall well-being. Exercise and engaging in hobbies can help improve physical and mental health, boost mood and self-esteem, and provide a sense of accomplishment and purpose. It's important to find activities that you enjoy and that are feasible for your current physical abilities and energy levels. Here are some strategies for staying active and engaged after treatment:

Consult with your healthcare team: Before starting any new exercise or activity, it's important to consult with your healthcare team to make sure it's safe for you. They can help you determine what activities are appropriate for your specific needs and can provide guidance on how to gradually increase your activity level as you recover.

Start slowly: After treatment, it's normal to feel tired and weak. It's important to listen to your body and take things slowly as you get back into an active routine. Start with low-impact activities, such as walking or yoga, and gradually increase your intensity and duration as you feel ready.

Find a workout buddy: Working out with a friend or family member can be motivating and provide social support. It can also make exercise more enjoyable and help you stay accountable to your fitness goals.

Mix it up: It's important to find activities that you enjoy and that keep you interested. Mixing up your routine with different types of exercise and hobbies can help prevent boredom and keep you motivated.

Take breaks as needed: It's okay to take breaks and rest when you need to. It's important to listen to your body and give yourself the time and space to rest and Recovery.

In conclusion, Chapter Six of The Cancer Journey Companion has explored the important role that exercise and hobbies can play in helping cancer survivors maintain physical and mental well-being during treatment and beyond. We have discussed the benefits of exercise and hobbies, offered tips for finding and maintaining an active and engaged lifestyle, and provided resources for further support. We hope that this chapter has provided you with the information and inspiration you need to stay active and engaged on your cancer journey. Remember, exercise and hobbies can be powerful tools in helping you maintain a sense of purpose and connection to the world around you. So don't be afraid to get out there and try new things, whether it's taking a walk around the block, picking up a new hobby, or joining a support group. By staying active and engaged, you can take an active role in your recovery and thrive during this challenging time.

CHAPTER SEVEN

Taking Care of Yourself: Self-Care Strategies for Maintaining Your Physical and Mental Health

Cancer treatment can be physically and emotionally draining, and it's important to prioritize your well-being to navigate this journey with strength and resilience. In this chapter, we will discuss the importance of developing a self-care routine, managing stress, eating well, getting enough sleep, and finding support

The Importance of Self-Care: Why it's crucial to prioritize your physical and mental health during cancer treatment and recovery.

The Importance of Self-Care for Cancer Survivors

Self-care is a crucial aspect of cancer treatment and recovery, and it's important to prioritize your well-being to navigate this journey with strength and resilience. Cancer treatment can be physically and emotionally draining, and taking care of yourself can help you cope with the challenges of treatment and improve your overall quality of life.

There are many different aspects to self-care, including physical, emotional, and mental health. Physical self-care involves taking care of your body by getting enough sleep, eating well, exercising, and managing physical side effects. Emotional self-care involves taking care of your mental and emotional well-being by finding ways to manage stress, practicing mindfulness, and seeking support from loved ones and healthcare professionals. Mental self-care involves taking care of your cognitive health by engaging in activities that challenge your brain, maintaining a positive outlook, and finding ways to manage anxiety and depression.

Self-care can take many different forms, and it's important to find activities and practices that work for you. Some people find relaxation techniques like meditation or yoga helpful, while others find solace in spending time with loved ones or engaging in creative pursuits. It's also important to remember that self-care is not selfish – it's an essential part of your recovery process, and taking care of yourself can help you feel more in control of your cancer journey.

One of the keys to successful self-care is developing a routine that works for you. This may involve setting aside specific times each day for self-care activities or incorporating self-care into your daily routine. It's also important to be flexible – your self-care routine may need to change as your treatment and recovery progress, and it's okay to adjust your routine as needed.

In addition to developing a self-care routine, it's also important to find ways to manage stress during cancer treatment. Stress can hurt your physical and mental health, and finding ways to reduce stress can help you feel more in control and improve your quality of life. Some stress management techniques include:

Exercise: Regular physical activity can help reduce stress and improve your mood.

Mindfulness: Practices like meditation can help you focus on the present moment and reduce stress.

Support: Seeking support from loved ones, healthcare professionals, and support groups can provide a sense of connection and help reduce stress.

Relaxation techniques: Techniques like deep breathing and progressive muscle relaxation can help you relax and manage stress.

It's also important to prioritize good nutrition during cancer treatment and recovery. Eating a balanced diet can help you maintain your strength and energy, and can also help manage side effects like nausea and weight loss. Some tips for eating well during cancer treatment include:

Eat a variety of foods: Aim to eat a variety of foods from all food groups to ensure you're getting the nutrients you need.

Don't skip meals: Try to eat regular meals and snacks to maintain your energy and strength.

Stay hydrated: Drink plenty of fluids to stay hydrated, especially if you're experiencing side effects like diarrhea or vomiting.

Manage side effects: If you're experiencing side effects like nausea or a decreased appetite, try eating smaller, more frequent meals or choosing foods that are easier to digest.

Getting enough sleep is also crucial for cancer survivors. Sleep helps your body repair and regenerate, and it's essential for maintaining your physical and mental health. Some tips for improving your sleep habits include:

Establish a bedtime routine: Try to go to bed and wake up at the same time every day, and create a relaxing bedtime routine

Make your sleep environment comfortable: A comfortable, cool, and dark room can help you sleep better.

Avoid screens before bed: The blue light emitted by screens can disrupt your sleep, so try to avoid screens for at least an hour before bed.

Avoid caffeine and alcohol: Caffeine and alcohol can disrupt your sleep, so try to limit your intake of these substances, especially close to bedtime.

Get regular exercise: Regular exercise can help improve your sleep but be sure to avoid vigorous exercise close to bedtime.

It's also important to seek out support during cancer treatment and recovery. Support can come in many forms, including support from loved ones, healthcare professionals, and support groups. Seeking support can provide a sense of connection and help reduce stress, and it can be an important source of strength and inspiration during this challenging time. Some ways to find support include:

Talking to loved ones: Sharing your feelings and experiences with loved ones can provide a sense of connection and support.

Seeking support from healthcare professionals: Your healthcare team can provide emotional support and guidance throughout your cancer journey.

Joining a support group: Support groups can provide a sense of connection and understanding, and can be a great resource for sharing experiences and finding support.

Finally, it's important to find ways to cope with the physical and emotional changes that can come with cancer treatment and recovery. These changes can be challenging, but finding ways to adapt and cope can help you feel more in control and improve your quality of life. Some strategies for coping with changes include:

Seeking support: As mentioned above, seeking support from loved ones, healthcare professionals, and support groups can provide a sense of connection and help you cope with changes.

Practicing mindfulness: Mindfulness practices like meditation can help you focus on the present moment and find a sense of peace.

Staying active: As discussed in Chapter Six, staying active can provide a sense of purpose and help you cope with changes.

Finding purpose: Finding meaning and purpose in your life can help you cope with changes and find a sense of direction.

In summary, self-care is an essential aspect of cancer treatment and recovery, and it's important to prioritize your physical, emotional, and mental well-being. By developing a self-care routine, managing stress, eating well, getting enough sleep, finding support, and coping with changes, you can take an active role in your recovery and thrive during this challenging time.

CONCLUSION

As you come to the end of this book, you may be feeling a mix of emotions. You may be feeling relieved that you have completed your cancer treatment, or you may be feeling anxious about what the future holds. No matter what you are feeling, it is important to remember that you have come a long way and have taken important steps toward improving your health and well-being.

You have learned about the various stages of cancer treatment, including diagnosis, surgery, chemotherapy, radiation, and follow-up care. You have also learned about the physical and emotional side effects of treatment and how to manage them. You have learned about the importance of maintaining a healthy lifestyle and finding support during this challenging time.

It's crucial to keep in mind that the treatment of cancer is not a one-size-fits-all solution. Your experience will be unique to you and will depend on many factors, including your specific type and stage of cancer, your treatment plan, and your individual needs and preferences. It is also important to remember that cancer treatment does not end when you complete your last treatment. Follow-up care is an important part of the cancer journey and will help you to monitor your health and manage any potential side effects or recurrence.

As you continue on your cancer journey, it is important to take care of yourself and seek support when you need it. You may find it helpful to connect with others who have gone through similar experiences, whether through support groups or online communities. You may also find it helpful to work with a therapist or counselor to manage your emotions and find ways to cope with the challenges you may face.

No matter what the future holds, it is important to remember that you are not alone and that there are resources available to help you navigate your cancer journey. You have the strength and resilience to face any challenges that come your way, and with the tips, tools, and strategies you have learned in this book, you can thrive through treatment and beyond.

www.ingramcontent.com/pod-product-compliance
Lightning Source LLC
LaVergne TN
LVHW010611160826
845677LV00013B/3365

* 9 7 9 8 3 7 1 1 8 7 3 4 5 *